Easy 20 Yoga Poses You Must Know As a Beginner (Yoga Poses for Stress, Anxiety Relief & Weight Loss) ™

Copyright © 2015 by Mia Conard

All rights reserved. No part of this publication may be reproduced, distributed, or transmitted in any form or by any means, including photocopying, recording, or other electronic or mechanical methods, without the prior written permission of the publisher, except in the case of brief quotations embodied in critical reviews and certain other noncommercial uses permitted by copyright law.

Contents

Introduction 3

Yoga Poses for Stress and Anxiety Relief 4

   Cat Pose (Bidalasana) 4
   Cow Pose (Bitilasana) 6
   Childs Pose (Balasana) 8
   Tree pose (Vrksasana) 10
   Extended Puppy Pose (Uttana Shishosana) 12
   Eagle Pose (Garudasana) 14
   Corpse pose (Shavasana) 16
   Lotus Pose (Padmasana) 17
   Hero Pose (Virasana) 19
   Legs up the wall (Viparita Karani) 21

Yoga Poses for Weight Loss 23

   Runner's Lunge Pose (Ardha Hanumanasana) 23
   Chair Pose (Utkatasana) 25
   Plank (Kumbhakasana) 27
   Garland Pose (Malasana) 29
   Warrior Pose (Virabhadrasana) 31
   Warrior Two (Virabhadrasana II) 33
   Inverted Triangle Pose (Parivritta Trikonasana) 35
   Locust Pose (Salabhasana) 37

Breath, Pose, And Connect - Adding Yoga to Our Daily Routine 39

Conclusion 42

Introduction

The book will be dedicated to easy yoga poses for beginners. Each pose will have a clear and concise list of instructions as well as an overview of what the body should look like at the end of the pose. The poses will focus on types that aid in benefiting the digestive system, encouraging weight loss, reducing stress as well as improving flexibility.

Yoga is a beneficial practice. Many people can be discouraged from trying it, due to a misconception that only bendy or flexible people are best suited for it. Women who look like they belong to toothpaste commercials with blinding smiles and slim bodies encased in tight forming clothes. Men who look like they can bend aluminum like rubber and arms and abs that make girls salivate. But yoga is for everyone. Of all sizes, builds, ages and skill levels. The great thing about yoga is its versatility. If a pose does not feel right, there are whole arrays of variants that are offered. So, don't be unnerved by yoga because you think you don't have the proper skills or don't have a "yoga body" and start your yoga adventure with this book.

Yoga Poses for Stress and Anxiety Relief

We have already discussed how yoga can be extremely beneficial at relieving everyday stress and anxiety. In this chapter, we will explore popular poses that will work at achieving this end.

Cat Pose (Bidalasana)

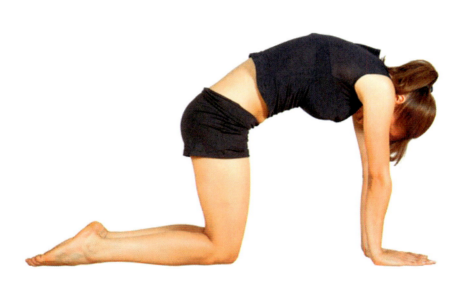

This is a great pose to include in the start of the practice, as it is especially low impact and gentle. Moreover, it is great for relieving stress and anxiety as you gentle curve your spine and hang your head in tranquility.

How to carry out this pose:

1. To begin this pose, move so that you are resting on your hands and knees. Check your posture, your hands should be directly under your shoulders, fingers splayed wide and your knees should be hip width apart. This is known as a *tabletop pose,* which will act as a starting foundation position for many poses. Move around and get comfortable, play around with this

movement. Rock side to side, stretch your limbs and take big deep breathes. Once you are comfortable and relaxed, you should move into the pose.
2. Inhale and exhale deeply and completely, through the nose. As you exhale, gentle round the spine and pull your abdominal muscles in towards the spine.
3. You should tuck your tailbone in as well as slightly tightening the muscles of your bum.
4. Push firmly down onto your mat with the palms of your hand as you increase the curve of the spine.
5. Your head should move downwards until it hangs limply down between your arms and you should bring your gaze to the floor.
6. The spine by now should be completely curved and resembling an arch or stretching cat.
7. Exhale and return to tabletop position. Repeat 10-15 times or as many as needed/wanted.

Additional benefits: Cat pose is also extremely beneficial to the flexibility of the spine, strengthening of the wrists and shoulders as well as toning or strengthening the abdominal muscles.

<u>*Posture check:*</u>

At start:
- Hands directly under the shoulders.
- Fingers spayed wide.
- Knees under the hips.
At the end or climax of the pose.
- Spine delicately curved, resembles a bridge.
- Head hanging limb and low between the arms. Eyes should be gazing at the floor.
- Palms pushing into the mat.
- Abdominal muscles drawn inwards towards the spine.

Follow up pose: Cow pose.

Cow Pose (Bitilasana)

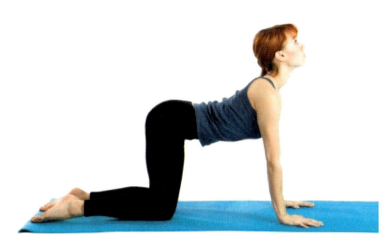

This pose is a great follow up for cat pose as they complement each other very well, and offer a nice starting sequence for your yoga session. Moreover, this combination of cat-cow sequence can be extremely calming and relaxing with its gentle movements accompanied by equally gentle breathing.

How to carry out this pose:

1. Similar to the cat pose, you should begin this pose in table top position. This means you should be on your knees and hands, with your palms directly under your shoulders and your knees under your hips.
2. Once you have come to this table top position, you can move into the cow pose.
3. Exhale and inhale, and on the inhale arch the spine gently and slowly, matching the breath to the movement of the spine.
4. As you arch your spine, you should press your palms into the mat, sink your belly down towards the ground and raise your head upwards. Your gaze should be straight forward and your chest should be facing outwards.
5. Exhale and return to tabletop. Repeat this movement 10-15 times, or as many as needed/wanted.

Additional benefits: Cow pose offers a gentle stretch to the neck and torso, as well as flexing and massaging the spine.

Posture check:

At the end of the pose:

- The spine should be dipped, gentle curving downwards.
- The tailbone should be raised to the celling.
- The hands should be spread wide and pushed into the mat.
- The chest should be facing forward.
- The head should be facing forward as well as the gaze.
- The knees should remain below the hips.

Best time to do this pose: At the beginning of a session, as it is a nice gentle way to stretch and warm the body.

Additional benefits: This pose is great to pair up with cat. This pairing is known as the cat-cow sequence.

Childs Pose (Balasana)

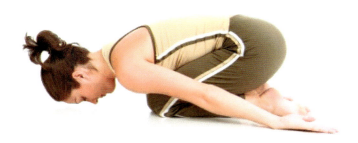

The child's pose is a yoga rest position that is optimal for the abating of stress relief and anxiety with its emphasis on breathe and stillness.

How to carry out this pose:

1. Begin by kneeling on the floor. The feet should be touching each other and the legs slightly apart and your butt should be released towards the heels.
2. Bend the torso forward so that it is touching the tops of the thighs.
3. Rest the forward on the floor.
4. Finally, move your arms so that they are resting comfortably ahead of your head on the mat or floor. Alternatively, you could chose to rest them backwards, facing back towards the end of the mat.
5. While in child's pose, you need to take deep inhales and exhales.
6. Stay in this position until you feel ready to move into the next asana. Though you should try to carry out at least 3-5 breath cycles.

Additional benefits: This pose stretches the muscles of the legs and back as well as the upper torso.

Posture check:

At the end of the pose:

- The chest and torso should be resting comfortably on the top of the thighs.

- The head should be resting, with the forehead touching the mat.
- The arms should be either positioned over the head or facing down towards the end of the mat.
- The shoulders and neck should be relaxed and not stiff or tight.
- Don't force this pose. If you can't comfortable rest your head on the floor use a pillow or block.

Best time to do this pose: Move into a child pose any time during a yoga session where you feel tired or a need for a brief respite.

Follow up pose: Any. Great to come into after a strenuous sequence as well as before moving into a difficult, high impact sequence.

Tree pose (Vrksasana)

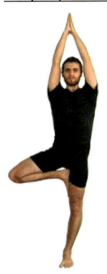

Rather than worry and stress, this pose makes you focus entirely on the art of balancing.

How to carry out this pose:

1. Move into mountain pose.
2. Inhale and slowly lift the left foot up from the mat.
3. Continue to bring the leg up, catch the knee with the hands.
4. Inhale and exhale. Find your balance by focusing on one point in the horizon. If you wish you can remain here, but if you feel confident you can intensify things a bit.
5. Bring the sole of the left foot to rest on the inner part of the right thigh. Find your balance. Lift your sternum up, straighten the spine and make sure the shoulders are away from the ears.

6. Press into the thigh and floor to keep balanced and for equal weight distribution.
7. Bring the hands together to either rest at the heart or have them raised above the head.
8. Stay for at least 6-8 breathe cycles. Release by bringing the leg and arms down.
9. Repeat on the other side.

<u>*Posture check:*</u>

- Spine straight.
- Gaze forward.
- Neck and jaw relaxed.
- Shoulders away from ears.
- One leg straight with sole of foot pressed into mat.
- Other leg bent with sole of foot pressed into opposing thigh.
- Sternum raised.
- Hands either by sides, clasped at heart or up above head.

Follow up pose: Any standing pose will be a great follow up to the tree pose.

Extended Puppy Pose (Uttana Shishosana)

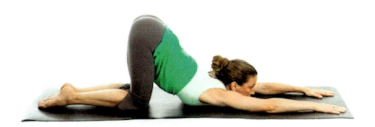

This is another gentle, relaxing pose that works to calm and ease the mind as well as the body.

How to carry out this pose:

1. To begin this pose, you need to come to tabletop position. The wrists should be in align with the shoulders and the knees directly under the hips.
2. Inhale and on the exhale slowly move the hands out towards the front on the mat. As the hands slide forward, the chest should be gently sinking towards the ground.
3. The knees should stay in alignment, directly under the hips, and the arms should remain shoulder length apart.
4. As you sink lower, gently place your forehead to the floor.
5. Firmly press the palms into the ground and as you do this gently lift your elbows and forearms off from the ground. Keep your shoulders relaxed and away from your ears.
6. Elevate your hips and tailbone upwards towards the ceiling.
7. Breathe deeply and gently stretch and lengthen the spine.
8. Remain in this pose as long as you wish. Once you feel ready to leave this position, lift the forehead from the ground and move back into tabletop pose.

Additional benefits: As well as being a great stress reliever, puppy pose is also immensely beneficial for the stretching of the spine, shoulders and arms.

Discomfort warning: If it is extremely uncomfortable to rest your forehead on the floor, then you can use a pillow or rolled up towel, which you can rest upon instead.

Posture check:

At the start of the pose:

- The hips should be stacked on top of the knees.
- The palms should be pressed into the mat. Weight should be evenly distributed as not to put undue stress on one of your wrists.
- The top of the feet should be resting on the mat.
- The shoulders should be in align with the wrists.
- The spine should be relaxed, displaying its natural curve.

At the end of the pose:

- The hips should remain stacked over the knees and the tops of the feet should remain resting on the mat.
- The hips and tailbone rose towards the ceiling. It should look as if you are pushing your bum upwards.
- The arms should remain shoulder length apart, the forearms should gently rest on the mat and the palms should also be pressed into the ground.
- The forehead should be lightly resting on the mat.
- The shoulders should be relaxed and away from the ears.

Best time for this pose: This pose is perfect for a gentle bedtime sequence as you release the stresses of your day. Moreover, as it is a partial rest pose you should use it during a sequence if you need to catch your breath.

Follow up pose: A great pose to follow extended puppy pose is downward facing dog.

Eagle Pose (Garudasana)

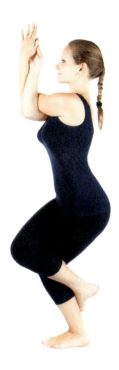

Because this pose requires immense levels of concentration, it diminishes stress and anxiety as you are forced to focus on the pose completely rather than the worrisome thoughts of the day. This is quite a difficult pose to master as it does entail balancing and using the strength of your body to hold this precarious pose. So if you are a beginner, you may find this pose to be a bit tough and involve a lot of falling over.

How to carry out this pose:

1. For this pose, you should begin in *mountain pose.* This position needs you to be standing up tall with the feet pressed together and the arms hanging down.
2. Breathe in and as you do, slowly raise the arms upwards until they are out in front. Think zombie arms. Next, gently wrap the arms around each other so that the palms come to be pressing together, facing upwards and the right elbow needs to rest in the left arm crease. If you can't get your palms to meet, then it is fine. Simply get them into a position that feels comfortable.

3. One an inhale, slowly lift your left leg and wrap it around your right leg. The left foot should hook around the back of the right leg.
4. Keep the hip and shoulders squared and facing forward, the shoulders down and away from the ears and the sternum raised. Do not let them tilt to one side, hunch to one side or hunch your back forward.
5. Remain in this position for a series of breath cycles. To keep balanced, you should focus the gaze onto one particular place or area.
6. Gently unravel your body, so you are back in mountain pose.
7. Repeat on the other side—lifting the right leg and wrapping around the left.

Additional Benefits: As well as aiding in the prevention of stress thoughts, the eagle pose is also extremely beneficial to the wrists, legs and hips, strengthening and stretching each.

Posture check:

At the start of the pose:

- Standing erect.
- Feet pressed together.
- Hands at sides.
- Head faced forward.

At the end of the pose:

- Shoulders down and away from the shoulders.
- Arms pressed together. One wrapped over the other with the palms pressed together.
- Leg wrapped around the other, foot hooked behind the other.
- Weight evenly distributed over standing foot.
- Back straight and long.

Best time for this pose: During a high impact yoga sequence that is focusing on strength and balance.

Follow up pose: Follow this pose with mountain pose.

Corpse pose (Shavasana)

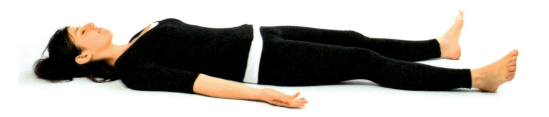

Nothing says peace and chill, then lying on the ground like the dead. This resting yoga pose is often used to conclude a yoga session for a period of silence and reflection.

How to carry out this pose:

1. Get situated on your mat by lying comfortably on your back.
2. Rest your arms gently by your side, palms facing upwards.
3. The legs should be long and relaxed, either splayed wide or close together. There should be no tension or stress in any part of your body.
4. Roll your head and neck, stretch the arms and legs, feel all the stresses of the day melt away as well as any pains and aches.
5. Inhale and exhale deeply and fully.
6. Stay in this pose for as long as it is desired.

Discomfort warning: If you feel any tension or discomfort in the neck area, place a rolled up towel or pillow under the neck or head. You need to be in a state of comfort for this pose, so make sure that you are actually are comfortable.

Best time for this pose: This is traditionally used to conclude a yoga sequence, so it is best to place it at the end of your yoga session.

Lotus Pose (Padmasana)

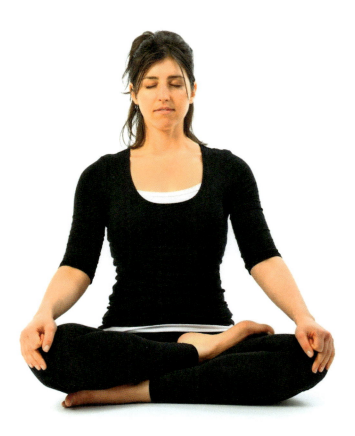

The lotus is an asana that requires the yogi to sit in a cross-legged position in a meditative state. The practice of the lotus is great for the reducing of stress as well as reaching a general calmness of mind.

How to carry out this pose:

1. Sit on your mat. Do not sit in any forced pose or position; simply sit in a way that feels natural. Take some deep, calming breaths.
2. Eventually come to a cross-legged position.
3. Once comfortable, lift one foot and position it one the opposite thigh. The sole of the foot should be facing upwards.
4. Lift the other foot and place it on the opposing thigh, with its sole facing upwards.
5. The knees should be down, touching the floor if able while the hands rest on the knees, open with palms facing upwards.

6. Breathe deeply and calmly. Try to keep stressful thoughts to the minimum, and focus on the body and breath. [1]

Additional Benefits: The lotus pose is extremely beneficial for the mind as it works at calming the brain, but it is also advantageous to the physical. This includes stretching the ankles and knees, contributes to a good posture and can actually aid in easing menstrual discomfort.

Posture check:

At the end of the pose:

- Feet placed on opposing thighs.
- Soles of feet facing upwards.
- Knees down, touching the floor if possible.
- Hands on knees, palms facing upwards.
- Head facing forward with the eyes closed.
- Relaxed jaw and neck.
- Torso and spine straight.

Discomfort warning: Some may find this sitting position uncomfortable, especially when attempting to depress the knees, which quite defeats the purpose of peace and calm. If you find your knees unwilling to touch the mat, then you can place a folded blanket under each knee.

Best time for this pose: This pose is great to do singular, apart from an entire yoga sequence. When you feel that you need to calm your mind, simply move into the lotus meditative asana. When doing this pose, as you should do with all yoga asanas, pick a space that is quiet and away from the noise and chaos of daily life.

Follow up pose: If you decide to include this in a sequence, you should follow it with a gentle resting pose, such as downward facing dog or a reclined twist.

Hero Pose (Virasana)

Acting as an alternative to the lotus pose, the hero pose is a resting asana that is splendid for the calming of the brain as well as the stretching of the limbs.

How to carry out this pose:

1. Kneel on the mat with your thighs vertical.
2. Move so the inner knees are touching and the feet are slightly wider than the hips.
3. The tops of the feet should be touching the mat, the soles facing upwards and the big toes turned inwards.
4. Stretch and straighten the torso and spine and lean forward. Move your legs slightly so your bottom can rest on the ground. The lower part of your legs should be resting beside your thighs. Once positioned, straighten the back once again.
5. Gently place the hands face down on top of the thighs.
6. Remain in hero pose for as long as you wish. Work to calm your mind and relax the body.

Additional Benefits: As well as working at calming the mind, the hero pose is extremely effective at stretching the knees and thighs and for improving posture.

Posture check:

At the end of the pose:

- The thighs perpendicular.
- The ankles and shins resting next to the thighs and hips.
- The hands placed down on thighs.
- The head facing forward, neck and jaw relaxed.
- The sitting bones resting on the mat.
- The soles of the feet facing up.

Discomfort warning: If you find this pose uncomfortable, you can place a block or blanket underneath the sitting bones.

Best time for this pose: Before you begin or during your sequence of sitting poses or before you begin standing poses.

Follow up pose: Recommended poses that work to follow the hero pose include the Seated staff pose, reclined twist or bridge pose.

Legs up the wall (Viparita Karani)

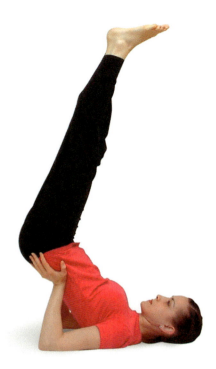

Who knew a wall could be so useful to the calming of the mind. But that is simply deemed as fact through this restorative inverted pose, which makes use of a wall and your pliable body.

How to carry out this pose:

1. Position your mat so that it is next to a clear wall. Choose a wall that is free from adornments, such as pictures and mirrors.
2. Arrange your body so that the left side is touching the wall.
3. Turn and place your legs up against the wall.
4. Your spine, neck and head should be resting on the mat and your bottom should be resting up against the wall. Use your hands to shift into position.
5. Moreover, your gaze should be skyward.
6. Inhale and exhale calmly. Stay in this position as long as you wish. Once you are ready to leave it, simply gently move your legs down the wall using the right side.

Posture check:

At the end of the pose:

- Legs straight up the wall. They should be straight and not bent.
- Spine, neck and head gently resting on the mat.
- Arms resting gently beside you. Palms facing upwards.
- Bottom touching the wall.
- Toes facing towards your head.

Discomfort warning: If you find this pose uncomfortable, place a pillow or blanket under the lower back.

Best time for this pose: Near the end of your yoga sequence, as it is a great pose to calm the body and mind.

Follow up pose: Corpse pose is a great pose to follow legs-up-the-wall, signifying the end of your yoga session.

Yoga Poses for Weight Loss

Poses to help with Weight Loss

Because of the relatively low-impact nature of yoga, its weight loss properties are occasionally marginalized. But they shouldn't. Yoga has been deemed as a suitable exercise that aids in weight loss as well as its effectiveness for firming and strengthening the muscles. Including only 3-4 sessions of yoga into your weekly schedule can dramatically alter your body, as it works at melting fat and toning muscle. In this chapter, we will present some popular yoga poses that are the most beneficial for those seeking to lose weight.

Runner's Lunge Pose (Ardha Hanumanasana)

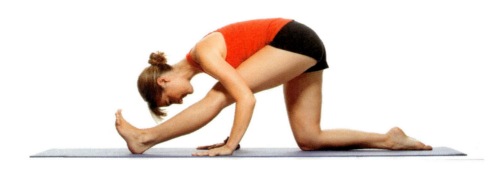

Get revved to go with this energetic pose.

How to carry out this pose:

1. Start in *downward facing dog*. See next chapter for instructions on that pose.
2. Inhale, and on the inhale bring your right leg up to rest in-between your hands. The knee should be stacked over the ankle and the thigh parallel to the mat. Your hands and feet should be in line with each other.
3. Your back leg should be posed on its tiptoes and still facing forward.
4. Distribute your weight evenly between the hands. Rise up slightly onto the tips of the fingers.
5. Stretch your neck and torso. Bring your gaze forward and your shoulders away from the ears.

6. Stay here for as long as desired. It can act as a quick transitional pose, where you only remain for a single breathe or you stay for 5-10 breathes, really stretching the groin and strengthening the arms and legs. It is up to you and your needs.
7. Release by bringing the leg back and moving into downward facing dog or plank, or rising up into warrior.
8. Repeat on the other side.

Posture check:

At the end of the pose:

- Back leg straight out behind. Facing forward. Weight resting on the toes.
- Front leg bent. Sole of foot pressed into the mat. Thigh parallel to the mat. Knee stacked over the ankle.
- Arms straight. Hands in line with the front foot. Weight resting on the fingers.
- Shoulders down and away from head
- Gaze forward.

Discomfort warning: If you feel uncomfortable carrying out this pose; simply let your back knee rest on the mat.

Best time for this pose: This is a great pose to move into after a downward facing dog during your yoga sequence. Moreover, if you are trying to make a sequence that strengthens the arms and legs then this pose will be a welcome addition.

Best follow up pose: Downward facing dog, so you can do the other side. Or warrior if you wish to rise up and start doing some standing yoga poses.

Chair Pose (Utkatasana)

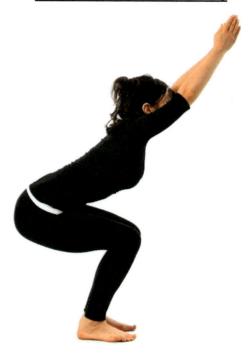

Sink down into this great pose to effectively tighten and tone the thighs, abdominals and bum.

How to carry out this pose:

1. Stand tall with the feet slightly apart and the arms hanging comfortably the sides.
2. Inhale. Bring the arms overhead while sinking the tailbone down towards the mat. To envisage this movement, think about sitting in a chair but without the actual chair.
3. Keep the torso long and the spine straight.
4. Inhale and exhale. Sink lower into this pose.
5. Stay as long as desired, aim for at least 3-5 breath cycles.
6. Inhale; straighten the knees rising back to mountain pose.

Posture check:

- Feet slightly apart.
- Arms raised and parallel to each other.

- Torso long and titled towards the ground.
- Gaze forward.
- Knees bent.
- Thighs should be as close to parallel to the floor as they can get.
- Knees over the feet.
- Tailbone sinking into the floor.

Follow up pose: Inhale and rise into mountain or carry out a balancing pose such as tree or eagle.

Plank (Kumbhakasana)

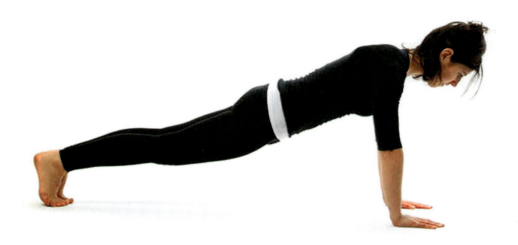

The plank can definitely be a workout for the arms. It pushes the yogi to hold their upper body up solely using the strength of the arms. Try this pose, if you wish to work on upper body strength.

How to carry out this pose:

1. A good pose to start in before moving into plank is *standing forward fold*. To find steps for this pose, see chapter four on *yoga poses for digestion*.
2. While in forward fold, press your palms firmly into the mat.
3. Jump or step back your feet towards the back of the mat. Position the feet so that you're on your tiptoes.
4. Keep your spine straight, the shoulders away from the ears and the palms firmly pressed into the mat.
5. Move your gaze downwards and keep it there.

Posture check:

At the end of the pose:

- Wrists and shoulders should be stacked.
- Hands firmly pressed into the mat.
- Neck long and jaw relaxed.
- Gaze downwards.
- Shoulders away from ears and shoulder blades spread.

- Spine long.
- Toes touching the mat.

Discomfort warning: If you experience strain on the wrists, you can lower your knees to the mat into a *half-plank*.

Best time for this pose: During a sun salutation sequence or after a forward bend.

Best follow up pose: Downward facing dog is a great pose to follow a plank.

Garland Pose (Malasana)

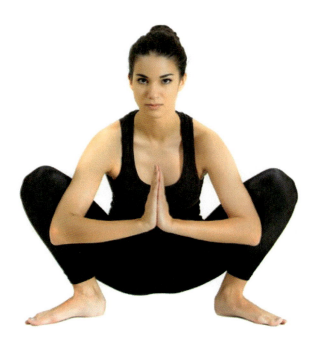

Squat down into this pose to tone and tighten your abdominals.

How to carry out this pose:

1. Squat down on your mat.
2. Press the feet together. Try to get the heels onto the floor.
3. Inhale and exhale. On an exhale, lean the torso down towards the floor. It should fit nicely between your legs.
4. Press the elbows into the inner knees. Bring the hands into a prayer formation.
5. Look forward. Keep on pressing the elbows into the knees as this will help you remain balanced.
6. Stay in this pose as long as desired. Try to remain in this pose for at least 4-5 breathes.
7. Release into a cross legged pose.

Posture check:

- Feet pressed together.
- Heels on floor. If this is too uncomfortable, you can remain on your tiptoes

- Knees wide apart.
- Elbows pressed into inner knees.
- Gaze forward or down.
- Torso tilted to the floor.

Follow up pose: This is a great posture to use for a transition from standing to sitting poses. Release this pose and gently move into a staff or reclined twist.

Warrior Pose (Virabhadrasana)

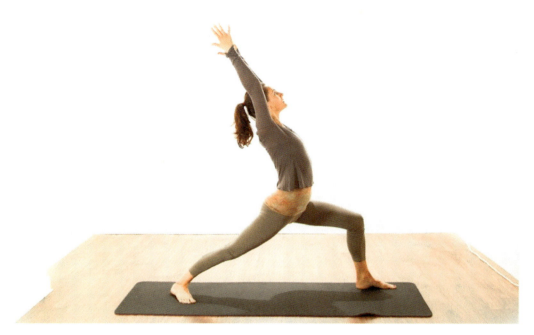

Be a warrior and conquer your weight problems with this engaging pose.

How to carry out this pose:

1. A great way to begin the warrior is by starting off in *runners lunge*.
2. From runners lunge, inhale and pivot on the back foot and rise up. Keep the front foot facing forward and bent, while the back leg will be unbent.
3. With an inhale, raise the hands straight up over the head. Keep the arms parallel, finger tips raised to the ceiling and next to the ears.
4. Inhale and exhale for at least 3-6 breath cycles.

Posture check:

At the end of the pose:

- Front upper thigh perpendicular to the floor.
- Front leg bent, knee should not be over the ankle.
- Back toes facing the edge of the mat.
- Back leg straight.
- Gaze forward.

- Arms raised, palms open with fingers positioned so they are facing the ceiling.
- Torso facing forward.

Best time for this pose: Warrior is used during sun salutation, but it is also great to use on its own.

Best follow up pose: Warrior two is a very suitable follow up pose, which we will describe next.

Warrior Two (Virabhadrasana II)

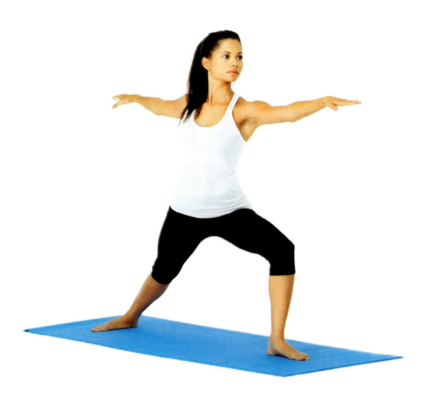

One a deep and calming exhale, move into warrior two from the previous warrior pose. Warrior two is very beneficial to the thighs and arms, as it draws on strength and balance to execute this pose perfectly.

How to carry out this pose:

1. First come to warrior pose.
2. From warrior, exhale and bring the arms from up overhead to parallel to the floor. The front arm should be out in front of you, in line with your gaze and your back arm stretched out behind.
3. Bring your gaze to the tips of your fingers or beyond.
4. Take 4-5 breath cycles in this pose, or as many as desired.
5. Repeat on other side.

Posture check:

At the end of the pose:

- Front upper thigh parallel to the floor.
- Front knee stacked over the ankle.
- Behind leg straight and turned towards the edge of the mat.
- Arms stretched and straight out so they are parallel to the mat.
- Gaze forward.
- Torso straight.

Best time for this pose: Warrior 2 is used during sun salutation, but it is also great to use on its own.

Best follow up pose: Inverted triangle is a very suitable follow up pose, which we will describe next.

Inverted Triangle Pose (Parivritta Trikonasana)

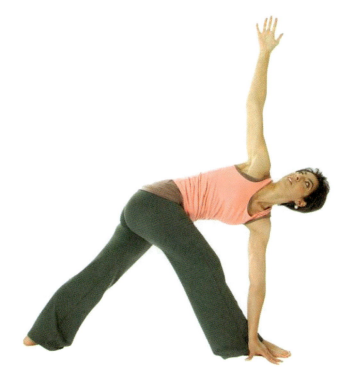

Ease down into this delightful yoga pose for a delicious stretch to the back, thighs, ankles and hips.

How to carry out this pose:

1. To initiate this pose, move into warrior then warrior two.
2. From warrior two, straighten out the front leg.
3. Inhale and on the exhale, slowly tip the body forward until the fingers or palm rest on the floor beside the front foot.
4. The other arm should be raised up above until it is facing skywards. Your gaze should follow this raised arm.
5. Stay here as long as desired, calmly breathe and relax into this pose.
6. Repeat on the other side.

Posture check:

At the end of the pose:

- Both legs straight.

- Front foot facing forward.
- Back foot turned at 90 degrees, facing the edge of the mat.
- Front arm straight, bent forward touching the mat or resting on the shin.
- Back arm risen over the head.
- Gaze up towards the ceiling, following the back arm's position.
- Torso long and stretched.

Discomfort warning: if you find it uncomfortable to rest it on the floor or shin, you can use a block to rest your hand atop.

Best time for this pose: Inverted triangle is a perfect pose to move into after warrior 2, but it is also great to use on its own.

Best follow up pose: A runner's lunge or a plank act as very suitable follow up poses for the inverted triangle.

Locust Pose (Salabhasana)

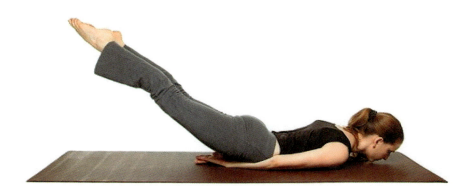

Far from being a pestilence, the locust pose is a weight loss blessing for the body.

How to carry out this pose:

1. Lie face down on the floor.
2. Rest your arms so they are facing the bottom or back of the mat. Rest the palms so they face upwards.
3. Inhale and on this inhale, lift your legs and chest up from the floor. Keep the legs straight as you lift.
4. Next lift your chest until it faces forward. Also lift your arms up; they should remain in their regular position. Facing the back of the mat, palms up.
5. Move your gaze forward and keep the neck long.
6. Stay as long as comfortable, calming breathing. Release on an exhale.

Posture check:

At the end of the pose:

- Legs straight out behind and elevated.
- Arms elevated beside the body. Palms faced upwards.
- Chest forward.
- Neck relaxed.
- Gaze forward.

Follow up pose: Bow pose is a challenging pose to try in following of the locust.

Breath, Pose, And Connect - Adding Yoga to Our Daily Routine

In the busy 21st century, when everything seems to be needed by yesterday and people go through their days in a whirlwind of chores, meetings, paperwork, classes and a million things more, the simple idea of connecting with our environment and with each other seems lost in the background; in the great era of fitness, healthy living, universal consciousness and wellbeing, the technology that allows us to share these ideas is the same one that has us playing the role of couch potatoes.

One day, we suddenly realize we can't move with the same ease, the normal chores we do every day seem more difficult and tiring, and we get sick or injured. We start looking at ourselves in the mirror and don't like so much what we see, but the mere idea of exercising puts us back to bed in the blink of an eye. We feel overwhelmed at the huge amount of work we have to put into it, and the million options we have for it: diets, weight routines, cross-fit, spinning classes, running, biking, swimming, and a really long etc. that gets us tired before we even start just by considering it.

On the other hand, when we finally understand our body's need to be cared for, cultivated and nourished, we take one or two of these options, and stick to them, with different degrees of success, or discouraging failures. We change those we don't like, learn to enjoy the ones we do, and the whole time we are looking for results and an overall feeling of wellness.

This is when Yoga comes in to do what its meaning in Sanskrit says, "to connect". We all know what it is, or at list have heard of it. Those of us who like to walk through a park have sometimes got a glimpse of a group of people standing or lying on 3x6 mats, stretching and bending in ways that defy physics, and wonder why in heaven they submit to what it seems to be a sophisticated form of self-torture. What we think is a masochistic behavior is, in reality, a set of postures, breathing exercises and meditative practices that has thousands of years and is recognized as one of the most complete exercise routines in existence.

The reasons why yoga has become increasingly popular are not easy to spot, but is self-evident that the practice has permeated at all levels in modern society. Whether yoga's popularity comes from pervasively high stress levels or stems from the recent trends among Hollywood stars, the many benefits yoga bestows upon its practitioners are easy to see (and feel). The American Osteopathic Association widely recommends it as a tool for increasing flexibility, muscle strength and tone, improve respiration, energy and metabolism, lose weight, improve athletic performance and develop protection from injuries.

However, there's one more benefit mentioned as the best of all things for yoga practitioners: it's an effective tool to manage stress, develop coping skills and a more positive outlook in life. This, in addition to the physical benefits, makes it one the most commonly used complementary health practices in the world, with very low risks associated to it when practiced under the supervision of a certified instructor.

Incorporating yoga to our daily routine will certainly benefit us in the short and long terms, but again, our busy schedules and several activities leave us very little time to dedicate to it. Nonetheless, there are ways to bring yoga into our lives, and here we list some of them:

1. **Wake up 15 min earlier for a Yoga short session:** Yes, we know, those last 15 min in the morning are perhaps the most delicious ones, but a short and simple Yoga routine, just before coffee, can significantly improve our energy levels throughout the day. There are several websites offering these routines, or you can ask your local yoga instructor at the gym.

2. **Incorporate it to your fitness weekly routine:** You can replace one or two of your sessions for a yoga class, use it as your "active rest" activity if you are into cross-fit or any sort of serious workout routine, or use it as your main activity if you are not doing anything. There's always a free class not 5 minutes away from home, and you can sign up for one at your local gym, if the monetary expense is a strong motivation for you to keep doing it consistently.

3. **Stretch:** Even in you don't like a formal yoga class, certain yoga postures and exercises can be used for stretching before and after your morning run, after long ours at your desk or during the heavy traffic at rush hour. Your muscles will thank you!

4. **Breathe:** In your car, your desk, the line at the grocery store, any place, you can take deep breaths and calm your body and your mind. This is one of the most important Yogic precepts, and one we can easily do anywhere.

5. **Meditate:** Take five minutes at the beginning or end of the day to relax, and focus only in your breathing, calming your mind and by it, making you more effective. A calmed mind finds ways around that previously are not considered or perceived, is more acute and efficient.

Yoga is not only a set of pretzel-like postures, it is a complete philosophy. It can improve our bodies, calm our minds, and make us better people, it deserves a shot.

Conclusion

Many people make the excuse of having too little time or being too busy for their reasons for not doing yoga. But the reality is that yoga only requires a small amount of time dedicated to its practice per day. Or you could even decide to do it every alternative day. It does not need to be done for hours; simply a daily 20 minute session of yoga can have a significant positive impact upon the body and mind.

To make sure you do include yoga into your life, make it part of your daily schedule or to do list. This could be in the form of a brief standing sequence during your lunch hour, an exhilarating morning session performed before you begin your day or a calming bedtime session. Yoga can essentially fit neatly into so many different times of the day, due to its versatility and lack of needed equipment. So, no more excuses about time or effort. Get started today.

The next step is to get practicing and gradually learn more of the hundreds of different yoga postures in existence today.

Printed in Great Britain
by Amazon